KELLY CLARKSON WEIGHT LOSS 2023

Inside Story of the Singer's Plant Paradox Diet That Helped Her Lose 40 Pounds

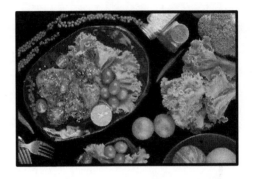

Laura Knight

TABLE OF CONTENT

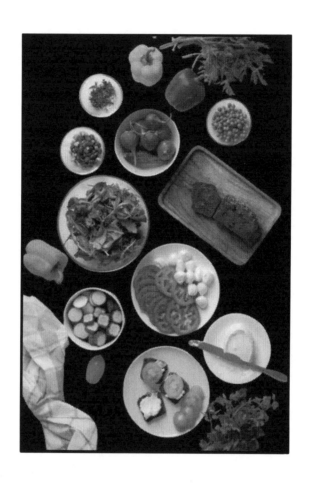

CHAPTER 1:

Harmonies Of Transformation

Kelly Clarkson, celebrated for exceptional singing and songwriting prowess, initially captivated audiences with victory on the inaugural season of American Idol. Transitioning into a successful career as a prominent pop and country artist, she has consistently remained in the limelight.

In recent times, however, the spotlight has shifted to a different aspect of her life—the remarkable transformation in her physique. Kelly Clarkson's journey toward significant weight loss has become a focal point of public interest, adding a new dimension to her already diverse career.

This delves into the intricacies of Kelly Clarkson's weight loss odyssey, exploring the pivotal elements that contributed to her success. Beyond the musical realm, her story serves as a testament to resilience and determination.

As fans and media closely observe her journey, Clarkson not only sheds pounds but also becomes a beacon of inspiration, sending a powerful message about body positivity to the world.

In addition to her musical accomplishments and weight loss journey, it's worth noting that Kelly Clarkson has also been an advocate for various social causes.

Her philanthropic efforts and vocal support for issues like education and equality further underscore the depth of her impact beyond the entertainment industry.

Examine Kelly Clarkson's weight loss journey, the contributing factors to her success, and the message she sends to the world about body positivity.

CHAPTER 2:

Beyond The Spotlight: Unveiling Kelly Clarkson's Weight Loss Symphony

Kelly Clarkson rose to fame as the victor of the inaugural season of American Idol in 2002. Since then, she has crafted eight albums, clinched three Grammy Awards, and assumed the role of a coach on The Voice.

The accomplished artist is also a mother to two children, River Rose and Remington Alexander, born during her marriage to ex-husband Brandon Blackstock.

Contrary to speculation about the use of weight loss aids like Ozempic, Kelly Clarkson's impressive weight loss of 40lbs took a different path. Dispelling rumors, a source close to Clarkson confirmed that she eschewed artificial methods, choosing a natural approach, as reported by OK!

The renowned singer showcased her transformed physique on her talk show, sporting a variety of stylish outfits.

In a departure from the trend of weight loss injections among celebrities, Clarkson embraced a more organic route—a disciplined diet and rigorous exercise routine.

According to She Finds, the 41-year-old artist consciously curtailed sugar and carb intake. Acknowledging her struggle with emotional eating, particularly post-divorce, Clarkson persevered in her weight loss journey, adhering to a health-conscious routine comprising a balanced diet and ample exercise.

The insider disclosed, "She's cut out soda, chips, biscuits, cheese and tortillas. And she's included regular exercise, largely cardio, into her weekly regimen."

Clarkson's commitment to change extended beyond simply changing her diet; she made regular exercise, especially cardio, a part of her routine. The result: was a significant weight loss of about 40 pounds, leaving her feeling rejuvenated.

Fans first noticed Clarkson's physical transformation in July, with insiders revealing a 15-pound weight loss. At that time, a source disclosed to Radar Online that she had embraced a healthy eating plan, emphasizing a regimen rich in protein while being low in carbs and calories. Clarkson's journey showcases her resilience and commitment to a healthier lifestyle.

CHAPTER 3:

The Healing Diet: Kelly's Path to Wellness and Liberation

Throughout Kelly's illustrious career, the media and public scrutiny have often targeted her weight, subjecting her to pressure and criticism.

Acknowledging her past, she revealed that she once succumbed to the unhealthy cycle of insufficient eating and excessive workouts in pursuit of a slender physique. Over time, she recognized the adverse effects of this lifestyle on her well-being and opted for a more sustainable approach.

Kelly's journey took a significant turn when she confronted health issues affecting her immune system and thyroid. Determined to regain control, she turned to the insights offered by Dr. Steven R. Gundry's book, "The Plant Paradox."

The book became a catalyst for her decision to adopt a lectin-free diet, emphasizing organic and non-genetically modified foods. In 2018, she underwent a remarkable weight loss of 40 pounds, attributing the transformation to her dietary changes inspired by Dr. Gundry's teachings. The shift wasn't just about shedding pounds; it was a medicinal endeavor.

Fully recovering from autoimmune and thyroid challenges, she proudly shared with Extra, "It was a transformative experience, and I am no longer taking medication."

Addressing the modifications in her diet, Kelly explained to Today host Hoda Kotb that the changes were not about sacrificing taste or familiarity. Instead, it involved using different ingredients while still enjoying favorite dishes.

This included opting for non-hormone poultry and alternative flours like cassava, tapioca, or almond. "The implementation of this process comes with a significant financial investment." She said.

In her journey, Kelly not only reshaped her physique but also found a renewed sense of empowerment, embracing her body at any size and prioritizing holistic well-being.

CHAPTER 4:

Understanding Foods Without Lectins

Lectins are proteins found in many plant-based foods like grains, beans, nuts, seeds, fruits, and vegetables. They help plants stay healthy by warding off bugs and diseases and might support our immune system too.

However, some people can be sensitive or allergic to lectins, experiencing stomach issues, swelling, or reactions after eating them.

The Plant Paradox diet suggests that lectins could be linked to various health problems, including being overweight, having diabetes, arthritis, and immune system disorders.

The idea is to eat fewer foods with lectins and more foods without, like leafy greens, broccoli, cauliflower, grass-fed meats, wild-caught fish, eggs, and healthy fats. This, according to the diet, can improve health and help with weight loss.

Kelly Clarkson followed this diet to address her immune system and thyroid issues. She didn't rely on workouts, pills, or supplements to lose weight.

Instead, she changed the types and quality of foods she ate. Kelly admitted the diet was a bit tough and costly initially, but she adapted and ended up liking it.

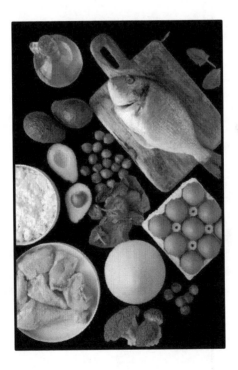

CHAPTER 5:

How Much Weight Did Kelly Clarkson Shed?

Kelly Clarkson successfully lost 40 pounds by sticking to the Plant Paradox diet. The noticeable transformation began in 2018 when she started appearing on various shows and events, showcasing a slimmer figure.

This positive change in her weight persisted until 2023, coinciding with the release of her deluxe album Chemistry and the commencement of her Las Vegas show.

Benefits of Kelly Clarkson's Weight Loss
By adopting a healthier lifestyle, Kelly experienced not just weight loss but several positive changes in her life.

Her physical and mental well-being significantly improved, resulting in increased energy, heightened self-confidence, and a more positive body image.

Notably, she shared that the diet played a crucial role in addressing her immune system and thyroid issues, eliminating the need for medication.

This transformation marked a holistic improvement in her overall health and well-being.

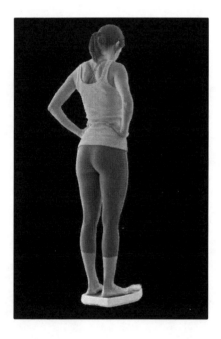

CHAPTER 6:

Kelly Clarkson's Divorce and Weight Loss Connection

Kelly Clarkson openly shared the profound challenges she faced in grappling with severe depression following her divorce from her husband and manager, Brandon Blackstock.

In an interview with "The People" for its Jan. 15 cover story, the 41-year-old singer revealed that she channeled her intense emotions into her most recent album, "Chemistry," a project that unfolded in the aftermath of her separation from Blackstock in March 2022.

The process of creating the album, according to Clarkson, served as her personal outlet for processing the complexities of her life.

She emphasized her disposition as a "let-go person" who does not harbor grudges, delving into a deep introspection of the events that transpired and contemplating her course of action.

Expressing her gratitude for having a healthy coping mechanism during the tumultuous period of divorce and grief, the Grammy winner articulated, "I cannot express how appreciative I feel for having that kind of healthy outlet.

Because the amount of despair and other issues that accompany divorce or grief are really difficult. You feel alone, and it's a blessing to have an outlet for those overpowering emotions."

The release of "Chemistry" marked a significant moment for Clarkson, symbolizing her reclaiming of power. In a candid acknowledgment of the therapeutic nature of the creative process, she shared her love for therapy, emphasizing its importance as a tool for navigating life and relationships.

Having recently relocated to New York for a fresh start, the inaugural winner of "American Idol" expressed genuine excitement about the unpredictable nature of the future.

She conveyed a profound understanding that life often takes unexpected turns, and the beauty lies in embracing those uncertainties.

In a parallel development, the interview coincided with revelations from a court filing, where Clarkson claimed that Blackstock, 47, once told her she wasn't "sexy enough" to be a coach on NBC's "The Voice."

This revelation shed light on the challenges she faced regarding her involvement with the show and Blackstock's comments about her suitability.

Despite the controversy and initial divorce filing in 2020, Clarkson eventually achieved her goal and became a coach on "The Voice" during its 14th season in 2018.

The legal proceedings also uncovered details about Blackstock's efforts to secure Clarkson a coaching position on the show, which led to a California labor commissioner ruling that he must pay $2.6 million to his ex-wife for unlawfully procuring deals that should have been secured through her talent manager.

Following her divorce from ex-husband Brandon Blackstock in 2022 with the resolution of that chapter in her life, she re-emerged onto the performance stage in Las Vegas at the Bakkt Theater of Planet Hollywood Resort & Casino with "Chemistry...an Intimate Night With Kelly Clarkson," debuting on July 28, 2023.

It's plausible that her energetic performances contributed to the noticeable changes in her physique during this period.

CHAPTER 7:

Is Kelly Clarkson a Personal Trainer?

In 2018, Kelly Clarkson made it clear that exercise didn't play a role in her weight loss. She humorously stated, "I am avoiding exercise! People may believe I'm exercising, to which I respond, 'Don't think I'm coming to play a sport!' Simply put, I haven't exercised at all."

However, after relocating her talk show to New York for the 2023 season, she found a way to stay active without hitting the gym. During an "8 Questions Before 8 a.m." segment on Today, she shared her approach to burning calories in the bustling city.
"In the Big Apple, walking is the most exciting aspect of life, " Kelly stated. She contrasted this with Los Angeles, where driving is the norm. Despite sounding unusual, her preference for walking aligns with the lifestyle change that came with her move. In Texas, where she spent considerable time, driving is the typical mode of transportation.

CHAPTER 8:

Kelly's Weight Loss Tips

Kelly Clarkson generously shares her wisdom for those on a weight loss or health improvement journey. These are some of her insightful words of wisdom:

• Do it for yourself: Kelly stresses that her weight loss journey was a personal decision fueled by the desire for a healthier life. She highlights the significance of self-love, encouraging individuals to find contentment with their bodies at any size. Her message urges people to prioritize their happiness over external opinions.

• Learn more: Before embracing the Plant Paradox diet, Kelly dedicated time to reading various books and articles on food and health. Finding valuable insights in Dr. Gundry's book, she recommends others do the same—learning more about nutrition and health to discover what works best for them.

• Be flexible: Kelly didn't rigidly stick to the diet, allowing herself flexibility. She enjoyed some of her favorite foods like wine, chocolate, and pizza but in moderation. Emphasizing balance, she advocates for savoring food without guilt or deprivation. Her approach fosters a healthy and sustainable relationship with food.

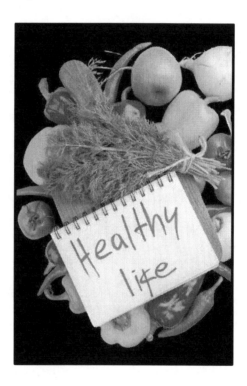

CONCLUSION

Kelly Clarkson's weight loss journey has captivated the public's interest. Her initial transformation, shedding 40 pounds in 2018, was credited to dietary adjustments, particularly opting for organic and non-GMO foods.

Kelly consistently refutes any use of diet pills or reliance on fad diets. While her divorce from Brandon Blackstock in 2022 might have influenced her weight loss, she clarified that exercise played a minor role. Instead, her active lifestyle in New York City contributed to maintaining her physique.

Kelly's journey sends a powerful message, underscoring the significance of health and well-being and highlighting the various paths to achieving personal goals.

For many seeking weight loss or improved health, Kelly Clarkson stands as an inspiring example. She demonstrates that by making simple changes in her diet, she successfully addressed health issues and achieved her weight loss goals.

Beyond physical transformation, Kelly radiates confidence and happiness with herself, embracing her size and shape. She generously shares tips for those looking to follow her example, emphasizing the importance of doing it for oneself, continuous learning, and maintaining flexibility. Kelly Clarkson's weight loss journey stands as a testament to the transformative impact of food choices and self-love.

Appreciation

I'd like to express my deepest gratitude to You for selecting my book, and I hope you enjoyed reading it. If you like it, would you please consider writing a review on Amazon to encourage others? I value your opinions as much as others seeking assistance with the same book. Your comments serve as motivation to me as an author. Knowing that my work has had a good influence motivates me to continue producing relevant and interesting content that appeals to readers like you. Furthermore, Whether your ideas focus on the characters, the narrative, or the general theme, they make a vital contribution to the book's journey.

Once again, thank you for choosing my book, and I look forward to hearing your thoughts.

ABOUT THE AUTHOR

Laura Knight, a passionate author dedicated to health and wellness promotion through her books, explores the transformative journey of **Kelly Clarkson's weight loss in 2023.**

Her cookbooks like "The Obesity Transformation Cookbook for Beginners" and "Intermittent Fasting for Men and Women with Obesity" showcase her commitment to wellness. With an adeptness for simplifying complex concepts, she also penned "The Anti-Anxiety Diet Cookbook", "30-Minute Heart Healthy Cookbook for Beginners" and "The Rise of Ice Baths Immersion.

Through her work, Laura motivates readers to embrace positive lifestyle changes via nourishing culinary experiences. Join her on a journey to optimal living.
For more advice and counseling, please write laurakthenutritionist@gmail.com

Made in the USA
Las Vegas, NV
22 May 2024

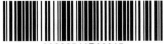